# THE ARMY INSIDE YOU
## A CHILDREN'S GUIDE TO THE MICROBIOME

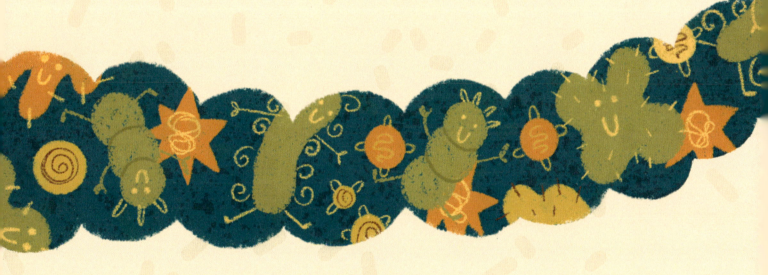

### WRITTEN BY
### LINDSEY GARVIN

### ILLUSTRATED BY
### BRISA A. GUERRA

~For all of the parents and caregivers, tirelessly working to raise healthy children in an unhealthy world.

**A Note to Parents and Caregivers:**

If you feel inspired to unlock the mystery of your own (or child's) microbiome, and seek to heal from the inside out, a functional medicine doctor or naturopathic doctor is a great way to begin your quest!

Copyright © 2022 By Lindsey Garvin & Brisa A. Guerra

All Rights Reserved

Published in the United States by Empowered Health Press

No part of this publication may be reproduced, stored in a retrieval system, or transmitted in any form or by any means, electronic, mechanical, photocopying, recording or otherwise without the prior permission of the publisher.

First published in America 2022.

# What is the Microbiome?

Your microbiome, or sometimes called the gut, is a collection of microorganisms that live inside your large intestine. These critters are so small that they can only be seen under a microscope.

Micro: small

Biome: environment

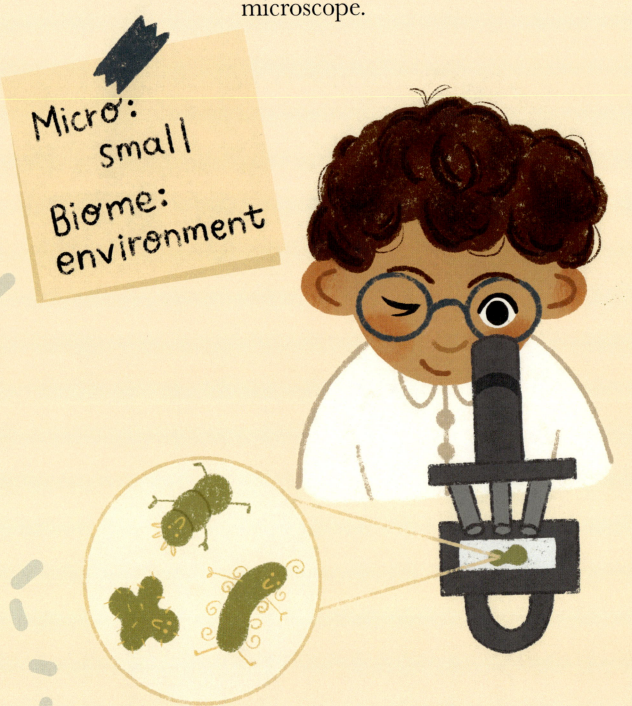

These living creatures make a home inside of you and have very important jobs.

large intestine

small intestine

Microbes live in almost all parts of your body, but over 95% live in the large intestine.

Did you know there are more microbes than human cells living inside of your body?

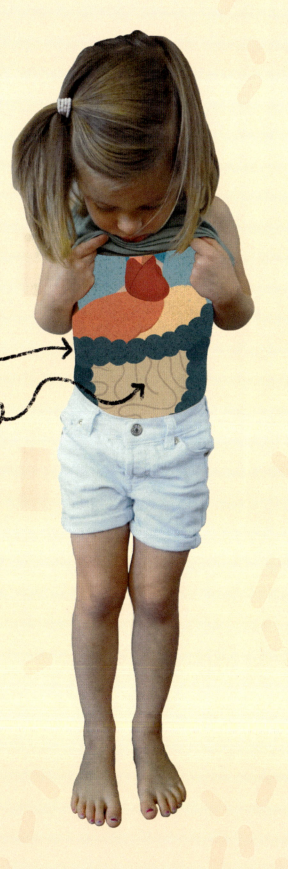

# Alive?!

Yes! These little critters are mostly bacteria, but can also include fungi, parasites, and viruses.

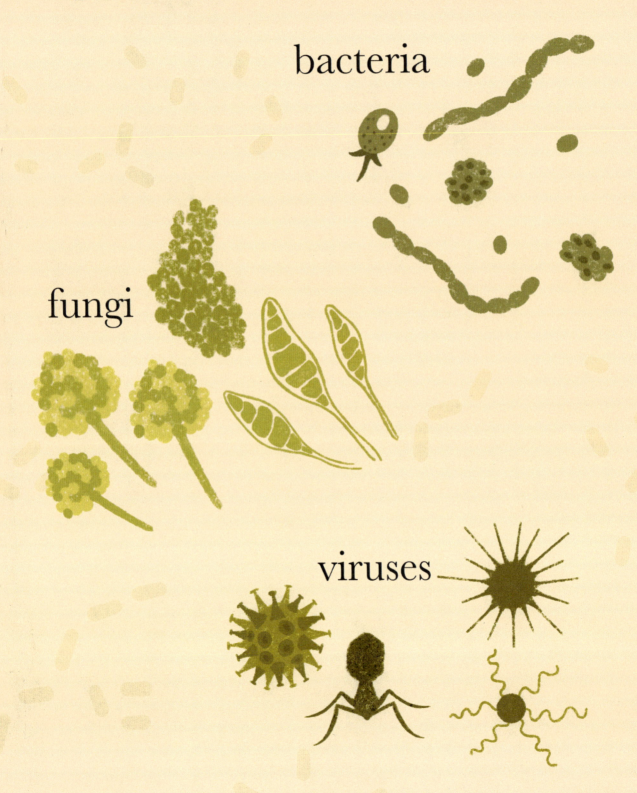

Not only are they alive, but they can reproduce, or make more microbes to grow into families and even cities of small species, all inside of your body!

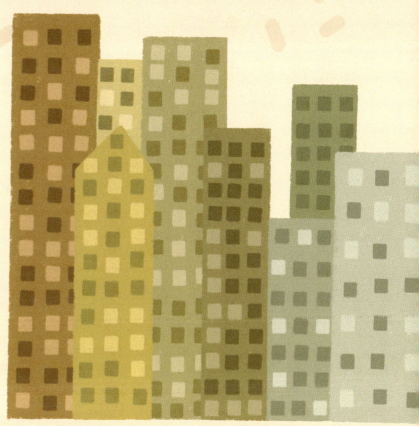

Reproduce: make more copies

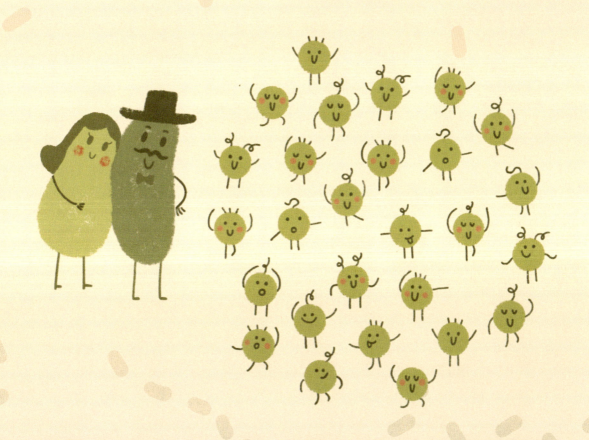

# Important Jobs

Our microbes do very important jobs for us.

Some help break down food, transforming it into nutrients to give us energy and help us grow.

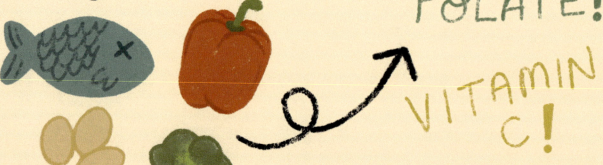

Many microbes help our immune system to be strong and fight illness.

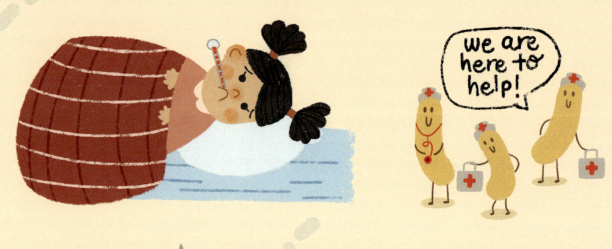

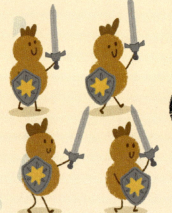

Some species are like soldiers that fight off bad microbes and toxins helping to keep us healthy.

What happens in the microbiome affects our brain, and some microbes can change the way we think and feel. They even have the power to change how we learn and remember.

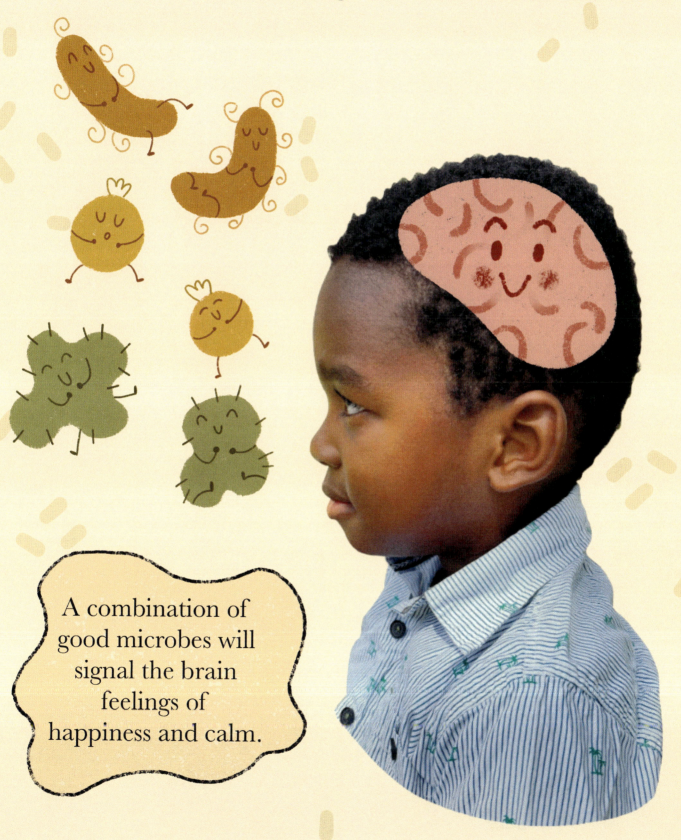

A combination of good microbes will signal the brain feelings of happiness and calm.

# The Problem

Some microbes can make you sick, or change your behavior, we call these pathogens. Pathogens are all around us. Some pesky microbial communities live inside us, and remain harmless in small numbers, but if they overgrow they can ruin the whole community of microbes, making us sick in all sorts of ways.

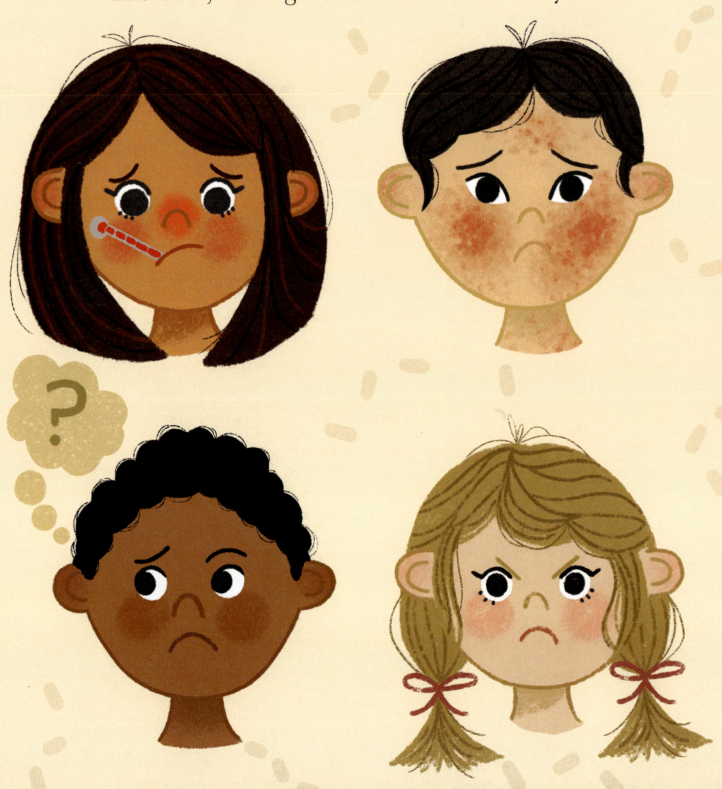

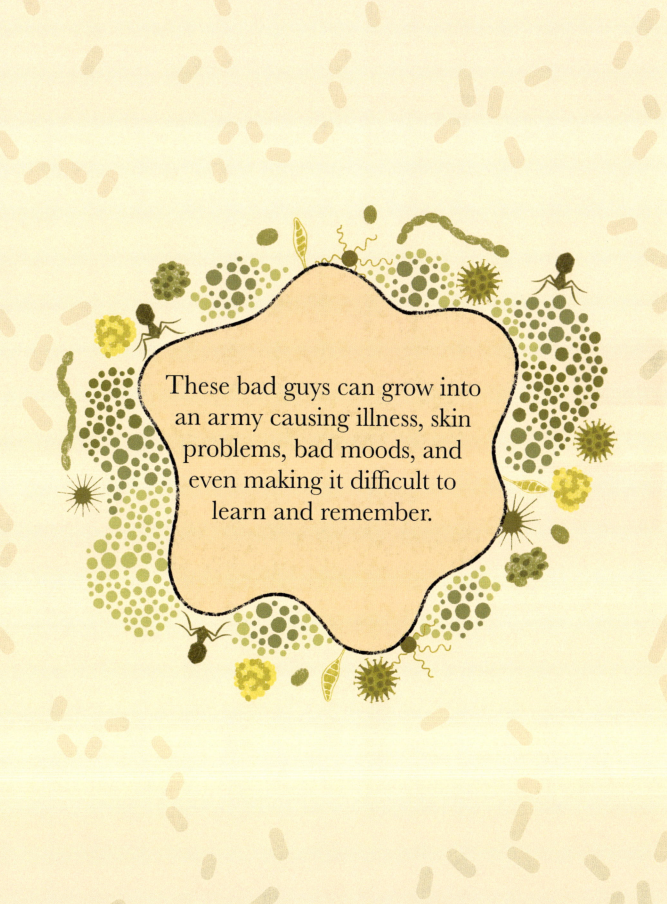

These bad guys can grow into an army causing illness, skin problems, bad moods, and even making it difficult to learn and remember.

# The War

Every moment our microbes are at war. The good guys are trying to kick out the bad guys, to keep us healthy. Meanwhile the bad guys try to grow and spread to overpower the good guys to make us weak.

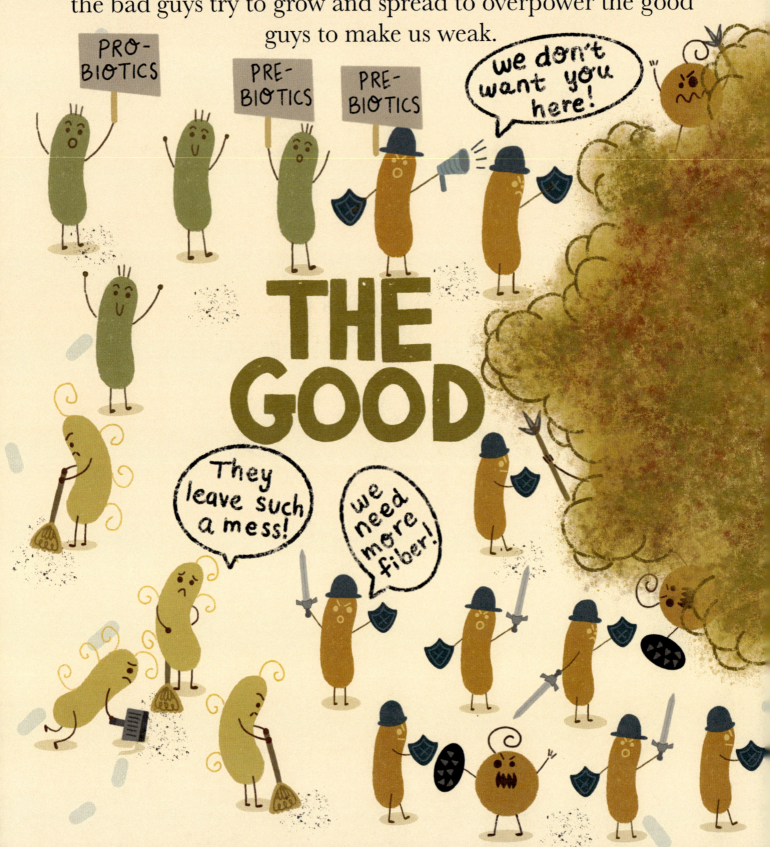

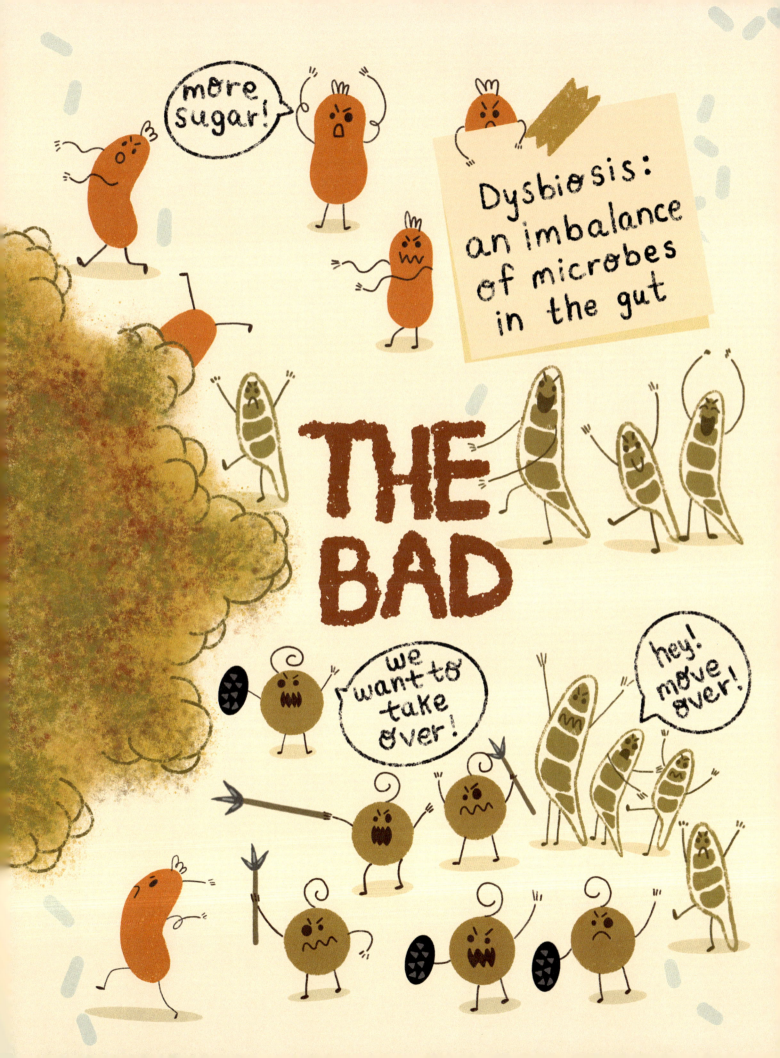

# You Can Help!

Every bite of food you take will either feed the good guys or the bad guys.

One organic apple contains 100 million diverse and healthy bacteria!

Whole, real foods, from nature are the best!

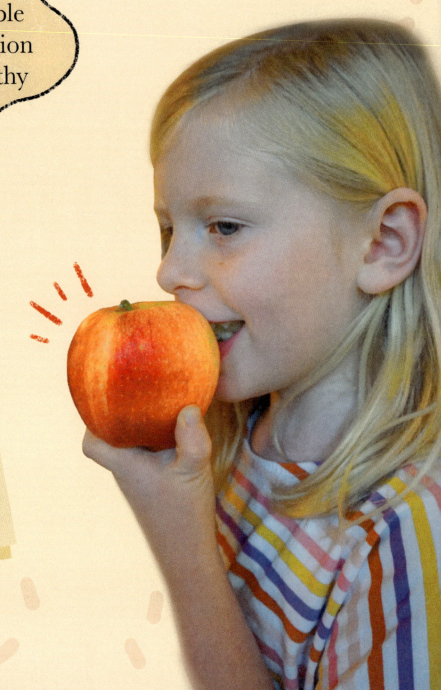

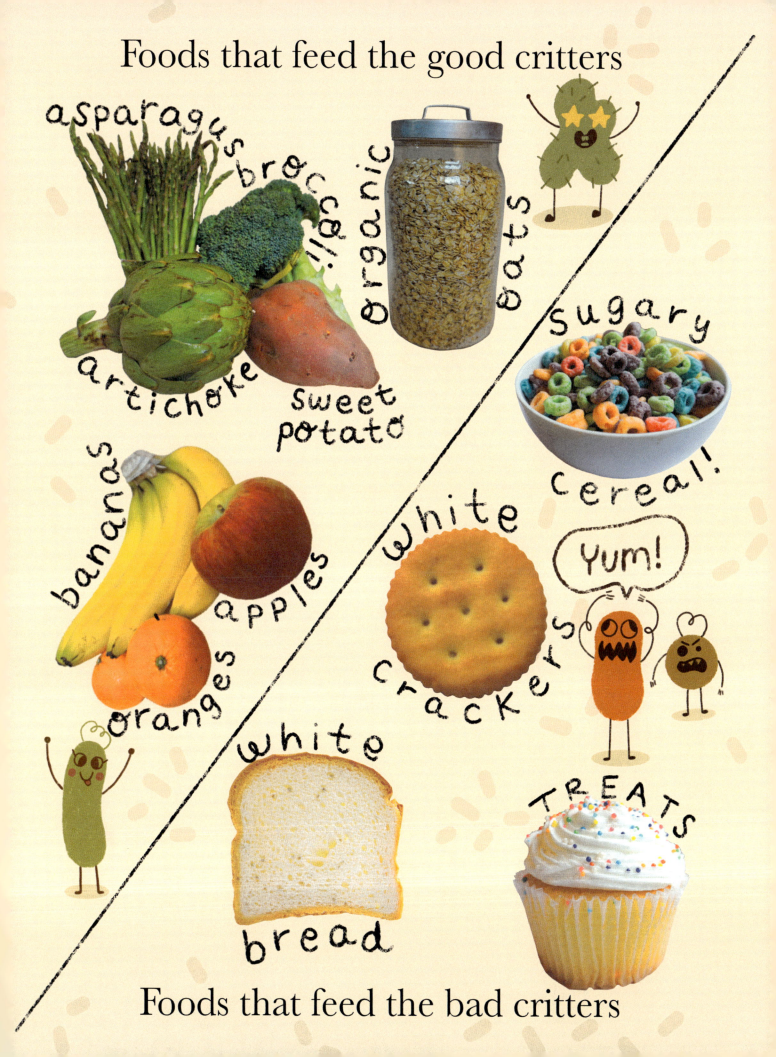

# The Sneaky Trick

Microbes are always trying to grow more of themselves. When bad microbes start to take over your gut, they can cause you to crave more of the bad foods that they love! This powers up the bad guys.

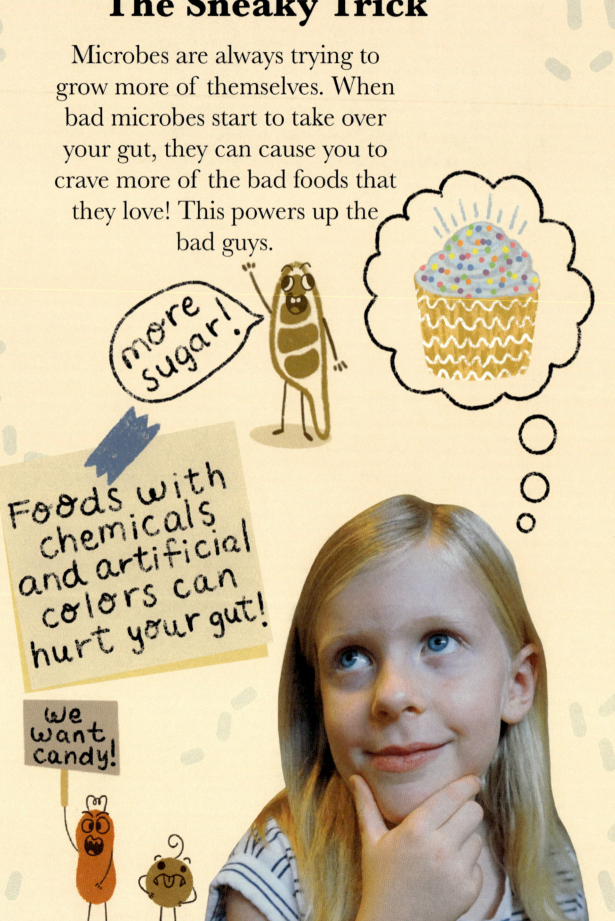

*more sugar!*

Foods with chemicals and artificial colors can hurt your gut!

*We want candy!*

Thankfully the good guys use this trick too. When your gut is filled with healthy microbes, they cause you to crave more healthy food, which feeds the good guys!

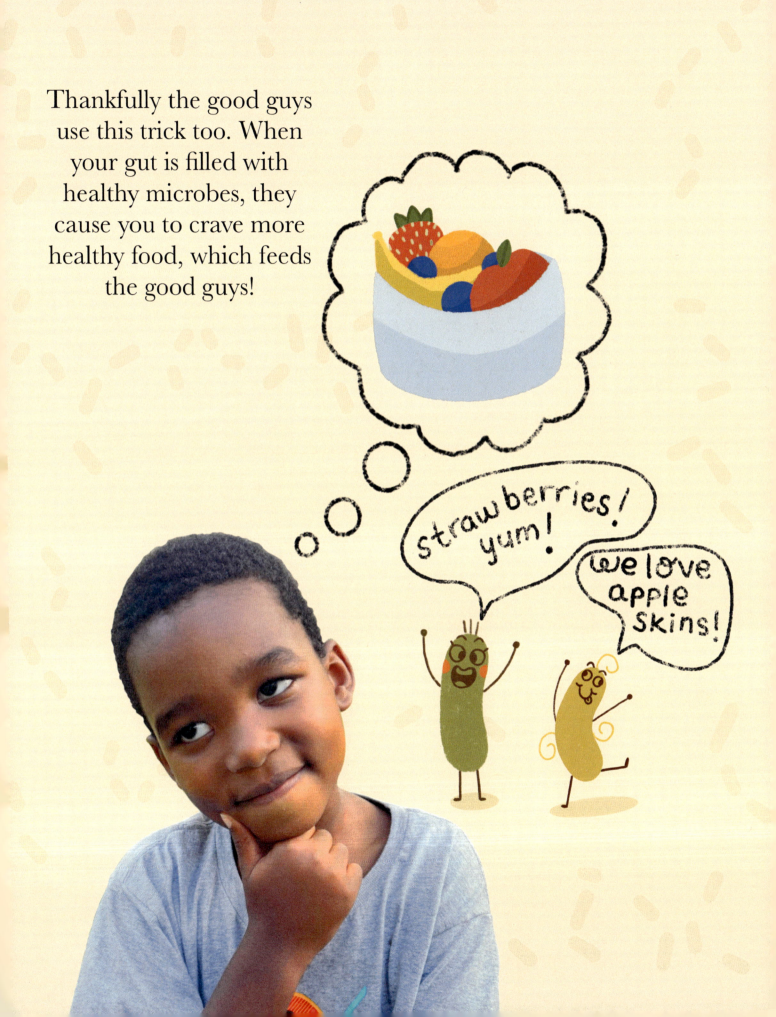

# Superfoods for the Gut

<u>Pro</u>biotic foods contain healthy bacteria that will make a home in your gut, adding to the good team, and pushing out the bad.

<u>Pre</u>biotic foods are fibrous foods that feed the good microbes, making them stronger, and their cities bigger.

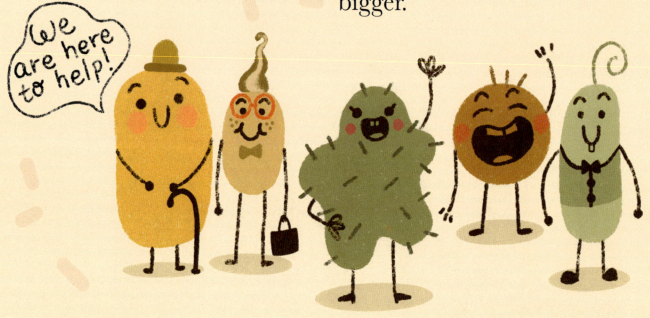

Fiber: The rough, undigistable parts of plants that the body cannot break down. Popcorn, fruit skins, berries, nuts, beans and veggies are excellent sources of fiber that will feed your good critters!

# Fermented Foods

Fermented foods are probiotic which means they are full of living bacteria waiting to make a home inside your gut.

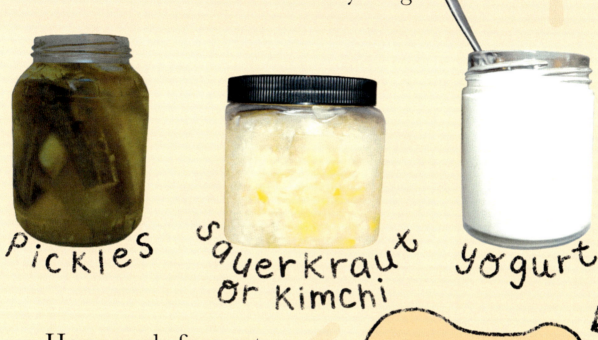

pickles    sauerkraut or kimchi    yogurt

Homemade ferments contain the highest amount of good bacteria, compared to store bought. With only 2-3 ingredients, it's easy to make at home!

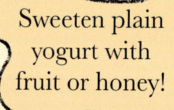

Sweeten plain yogurt with fruit or honey!

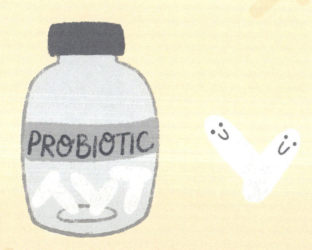

Sometimes an adult may give you probiotics as a pill or powder!

# A Healthy Microbiome

By eating whole, real foods that feed your good guys you will create a healthy habitat for your microbes to flourish and keep you healthy.

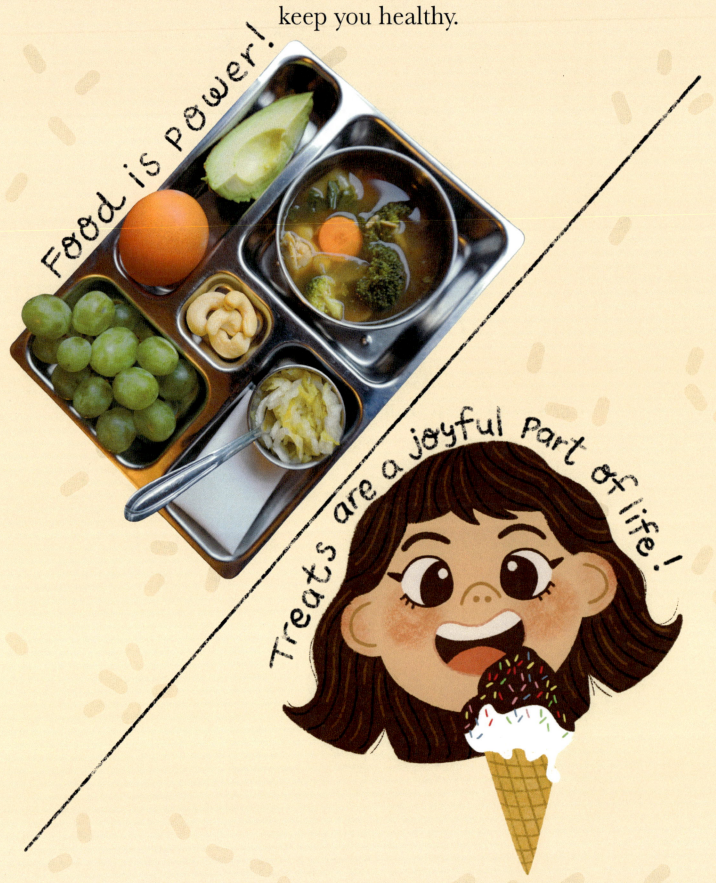

Food is power!

Treats are a joyful part of life!

That way an occasional treat won't stand a chance at starting a war with the good guys.

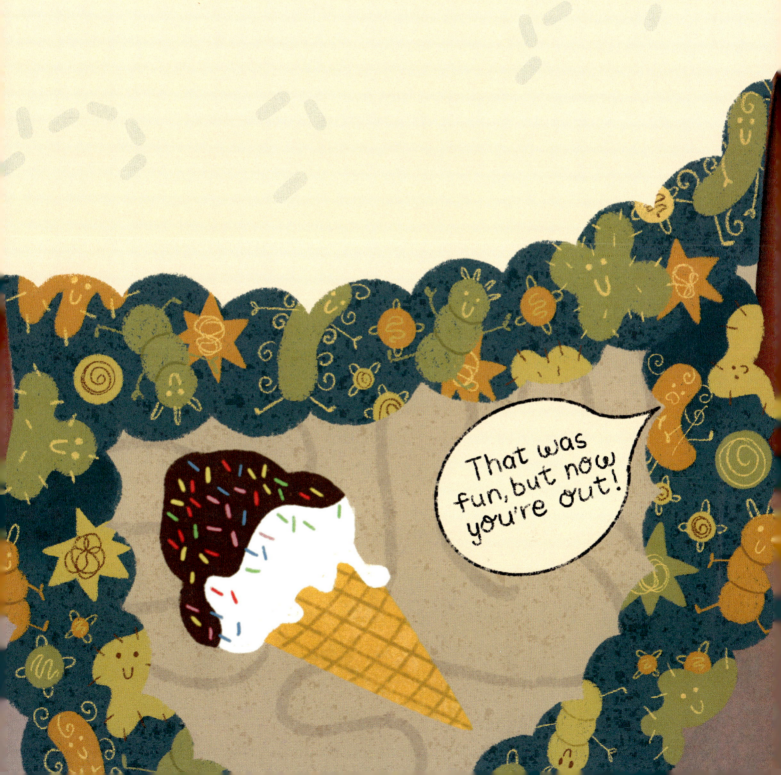

# Other Amazing Food Choices for a Happy Microbiome

- Cucumbers
- Carrots
- Bell Peppers
- Leafy greens
- Pomegranate
- Pears
- Onions
- Garlic
- Jicama
- Tomatoes
- Avocados
- Mushrooms

- Not-yet-ripe bananas
- Fresh or dried herbs
- Berries (frozen or fresh)
- Homemade sourdough bread
- Organic wheat and seeded bread
- Quinoa
- Pumpkin seeds
- Chia seeds
- Grass-fed and organic meats
- Coconut, avocado and olive oils
- Bone broth
- Wild caught fish

*Your microbes love it when you try new foods!*

# Gut Healthy Snack Ideas

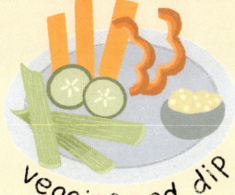
veggies and dip

Must Contain:
1. Fiber
2. Vitamins/Minerals

apples and nut butter or sunflower seed butter

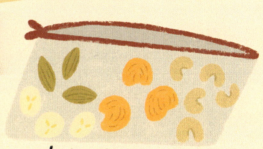
dried fruit and nuts

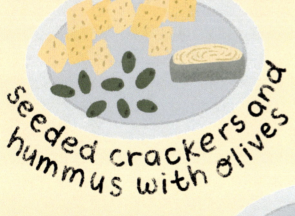
seeded crackers and hummus with olives

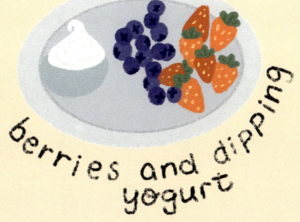
berries and dipping yogurt

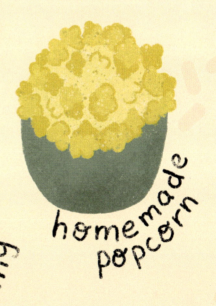
homemade popcorn

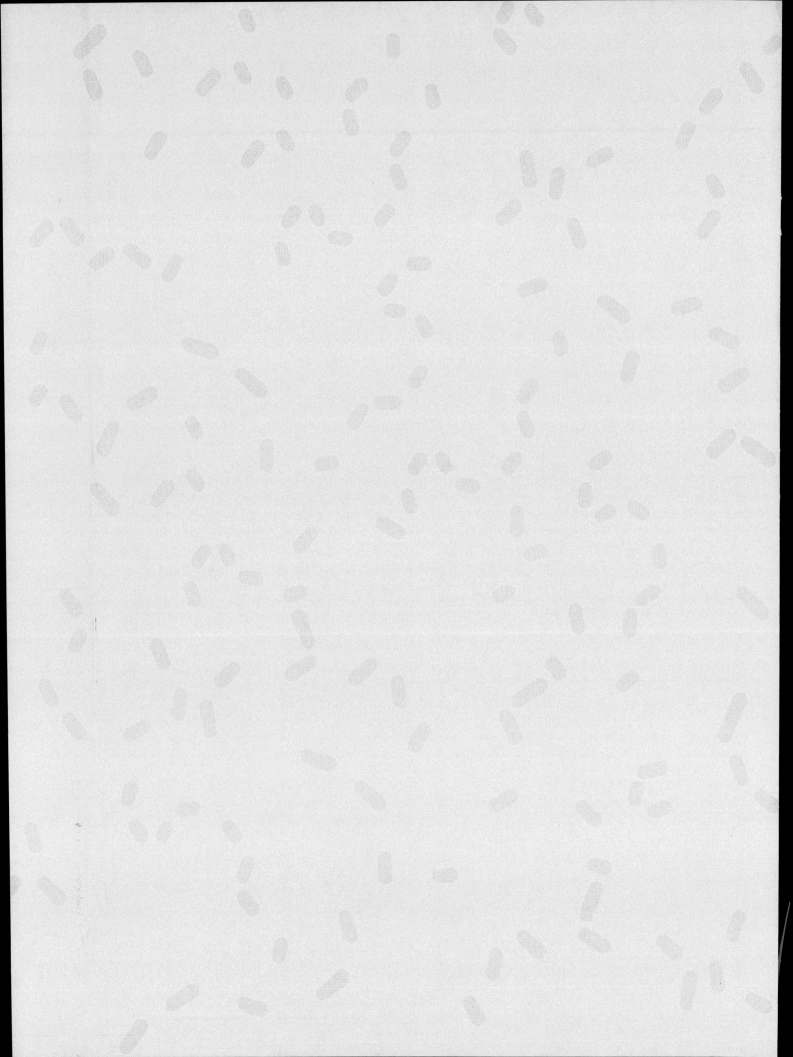